I've Been Diagnosed with PCOS, Now What?

A Guide to Thriving with Polycystic Ovary Syndrome

By Lisa A. Borunda Conner, FNP-BC

Table of Contents

Acknowledgements ii

Introduction...iii

Chapter 1: What is PCOS/Why is it Important to Treat 1
    Identifying PCOS...1
    Myths about PCOS 2
    Importance of Diagnosing and Treating PCOS...2

Chapter 2: Diagnosing PCOS 4
    Diagnostic Criteria...4
    History and Physical for Diagnosis 4
    Ultrasound 4
    Laboratory Tests 5

Chapter 3: Role of Insulin Resistance and Elevated Androgens...........................7
    Signs and Symptoms of Insulin Resistance..7
    Acanthosis Nigricans...7
    How Insulin Resistance Develops..8
    Seven Ways to Treat Insulin Resistance 8
    Insulin Resistance Syndrome (AKA Metabolic Syndrome) 9
    Waist-to-Hip Ratio...10

Chapter 4: Treating PCOS...11
    AACE Treatment Guidelines..11
    Medications 12
    Exercise/weight loss 14

Chapter 5: Infertility...15

Chapter 6: Psychological Aspects of PCOS 17
    Eating Disorders and Altered Body Image.. 17

Chapter 7: PCOS Education...19
    FAQ Handout..19
    PCOS Basics Handout 19
    Nutritional Handouts...19

Chapter 8: Multidisciplinary Approach to Care 20

Chapter 9: PCOS Support Group and Success Stories 21

Chapter 10: PCOS Resources, Apps and OnlineSupport.....................................24
    Resources 24
    Apps and Online Support...24

Appendix A: Glossary of Terms 25

Appendix B: Diagnostic Criteria... 27

Appendix C: Habit Change Cheat Sheet.. 28

Appendix D: U.S. Health and Human Services PCOS FAQ...................................31

Appendix E: Sample of PCOS Basics Handout 37

Notes/Questions for Healthcare Provider...38

References.. 39

Acknowledgements

I want to thank my wonderful husband, Rex Conner, for his encouragement to write my second book and share this information on a much larger scale than could be accomplished in the clinic alone. I love our life!

I want to thank our children, family, friends, and coworkers for their constant love and encouragement.

I also want to thank my wonderful employers and friends, Dr. Chad and Diana Lunt.

I especially want to thank all of my patients for believing in me and entrusting their care to me.

Introduction

My previous book *How to Build a Strong PCOS Practice, Treating One Beautiful Woman at a Time* was written for healthcare providers. This, my second book, is for people affected by PCOS, whether you personally have PCOS or a friend or loved one does.

A common condition affecting approximately 10 percent of women, PCOS is complex, but it doesn't have to be complicated. If you learn all you can about it and get the right treatment and support, then you will live a happier, healthier life.

The PCOS treatment helps you to lose weight, decrease insulin levels, balance hormones, improve fertility, regulate cycles, and decrease the risk of long-term health complications. A combination of exercise, healthy eating, medication, and/or supplements may be used to treat the condition.

Maybe you were motivated to seek treatment for PCOS because of a specific problem like weight gain, dark hair growth, or difficulty getting pregnant. As you initiate treatment, you will find more benefits to your health and well-being than you ever expected.

In the short run, you will feel better because you will have fewer PCOS symptoms (fatigue, sugar cravings, dark hair growth, acne, mood swings, bleeding irregularities, weight gain, and so on). Your long-term health will also benefit because you will decrease your odds of developing diabetes, high blood pressure, heart disease, and other health complications.

I hope this guide will inspire you to do everything you can to proactively treat PCOS. When you treat PCOS you will feel and look better and people will ask you what you are doing. Take the opportunity to educate others about PCOS and be an advocate within your own family and community. You will likely have many opportunities to share your knowledge and your personal success story. Just remember, PCOS is manageable with the right treatment and support!

Best Wishes,

Lisa A. Borunda Conner, FNP-BC

Chapter 1: What is PCOS/Why is it Important to Treat

What is PCOS

Polycystic Ovary Syndrome (PCOS) is a common hormonal disorder that affects approximately 10 percent of reproductive age women—around 5 million women in the United States.

A polycystic ovary has multiple small "cysts," which are actually small follicles that stopped developing due to a hormonal imbalance. When a follicle develops but does not reach full maturity (and fails to release an egg) the remnant of the follicle may remain along the edge of the ovary. Women who have PCOS secrete higher than normal amounts of male hormones (mainly testosterone), but polycystic ovaries are a symptom of a hormonal imbalance not the cause.

Although PCOS is a common cause of infertility, it also has the potential to affect multiple systems of the body and can increase a woman's risk for emotional and physical health problems.

As if dealing with the symptoms of PCOS wasn't enough, PCOS also increases a woman's risk for diseases such as type 2 diabetes and heart disease. That's why treating PCOS is so important.

Many women suffer with the symptoms of PCOS for years without ever receiving a diagnosis. The fact that you have received a diagnosis and are starting treatment is positive! Many women see multiple specialists for symptoms of PCOS, and far too often the pieces aren't pulled together to make the diagnosis and PCOS is missed or misdiagnosed.

Passed down genetically, PCOS requires only one parent to be a carrier for the child to inherit the predisposing gene, and each pregnancy has a 50 percent chance of carrying the abnormal gene. However, not all people who inherit the gene will develop PCOS. Men may be carriers of PCOS. They may have no symptoms or have symptoms such as early baldness and excessive hair growth. They are more likely to gain weight in their abdomen and are at higher risk for insulin resistance, type 2 diabetes, and heart problems.

PCOS was first recognized in 1935 as Stein-Leventhal syndrome (named after the two American physicians who discovered the relationship between multiple follicles on the ovaries and irregular menstrual cycles). However, the first PCOS textbook was not written until 1984 by an expert named Walter Futterweit, M.D. Furthermore, the link between insulin resistance and PCOS was not discovered until the 1990s. The medication Metformin, which is commonly used to treat insulin resistance in type 2 diabetes and PCOS, has only been on the market in the United States since 1995. We are learning more about PCOS all the time.

Identifying PCOS

As previously mentioned, identifying PCOS remains a major challenge and most women see several health care providers before receiving a diagnosis. They often seek treatment from multiple specialists for the symptoms of PCOS. For example, a woman may seek treatment from a dermatologist for acne and a gynecologist for irregular cycles. Seeing multiple specialists can fragment care, and although each specialist manages the symptoms specific to his or her area of expertise, PCOS can be easily missed.

I have seen patients who have been told they have elevated testosterone and insulin resistance and are being treated for both, but they have never heard of PCOS. I think it's important to call it what it is so people can learn about the intricacies of PCOS and treat the whole syndrome.

Note: If a woman starts on birth control for irregular cycles without having a proper work-up, she may be led to believe that birth control cured her irregular cycles. Additionally, she may have no idea that she may have a condition that could affect her weight, fertility, and significantly increase her risk for type 2 diabetes, heart disease, and other long-term health problems. Up to 80 percent of women with irregular cycles have PCOS.

Myths about PCOS

The following myths have persisted for decades about this condition:

- ❖ You are too thin to have PCOS. (Fact: only 60 to 70 percent of women with PCOS are overweight.)

- ❖ You do not have PCOS because you have had children. (Fact: many women with PCOS ovulate intermittently and conceive spontaneously; many others conceive with the help of assisted reproduction.)

- ❖ If you eat less and exercise more, you'll lose weight. (Fact: that is true for many but not all women with PCOS. Sometimes it has a whole lot more to do with **what** they eat. Insulin resistance can make weight loss difficult. Ask for a referral to a dietician for help with personalized meal planning for insulin resistance/PCOS).

- ❖ You do not have PCOS because your testosterone level is normal. (Fact: many women do not have elevated circulating androgens such as testosterone. Clinical evidence of androgen excess such as dark hair growth on the face and body also meets the criteria for PCOS.)

- ❖ You must have polycystic appearing ovaries, on ultrasound, to have PCOS. (Fact: only 75 percent of women with PCOS will have polycystic ovaries.)

- ❖ If you cycle regularly you do not have PCOS. (Fact: some women with PCOS have regular cycles. Many others do not understand that cycles of fewer than 21 days or more than 35 days apart are not considered regular).

Importance of Diagnosing and Treating PCOS

Let me emphasize why it is so important to diagnose and properly treat PCOS. PCOS can greatly affect a person's quality of life and significantly increase the risk for other conditions.

According to the US Department of Health and Human Services, Office on Women's Health, more than 50 percent of women with PCOS will have impaired glucose tolerance (pre-diabetes) or type 2 diabetes before the age of 40. They also have a 4 to 7 times greater risk of heart attack than their same-aged peers without PCOS.

In addition, they may suffer from one or many of the additional symptoms and conditions associated with PCOS, such as:

- ❖ obesity
- ❖ premenstrual syndrome (PMS)
- ❖ depression
- ❖ anxiety
- ❖ acne
- ❖ abnormal dark hair growth on face and body
- ❖ male pattern baldness
- ❖ sleep apnea
- ❖ thyroid problems
- ❖ non-alcoholic fatty liver disease (NAFLD)
- ❖ recurrent miscarriage
- ❖ infertility
- ❖ endometrial hyperplasia or pre-cancer
- ❖ cancer of the uterus
- ❖ elevated cholesterol and triglycerides
- ❖ high blood pressure.

Chapter 2: Diagnosing PCOS

Diagnostic Criteria

There are three different criteria for diagnosing PCOS (see Appendix B). They vary slightly and require either two or three of the following:

1. Irregular cycles
2. Signs of elevated androgens (such as high testosterone or dark hair growth)
3. Polycystic ovaries.

History and Physical for Diagnosis

A detailed history is important to diagnosing PCOS. Many conditions occur throughout a woman's life that can tip off doctors about this condition. Let's look at some of these possible conditions in a woman's health history.

One common condition is irregular or absent menstrual periods. These usually begin in the teen years, but frequently people with PCOS have started birth control as teens, and the diagnosis of PCOS is not made until they try to conceive in their twenties or later. Often cycles are 35 days or more apart. Some women skip months, while others have continuous spotting or more than one period a month.

These irregular cycles can become a problem later in life. Some women report regular cycles and no difficulty conceiving their first child or two and then things change: cycles become irregular, they stop ovulating, and their infertility work-up leads to a PCOS diagnosis.

Two conditions that could signal PCOS relate to clinical (physical) symptoms of androgen excess: male pattern hair growth (dark hair growth on the face and body) and acne. For androgens to have an effect on the skin they must bind with a skin androgen receptor and have adequate enzyme converting capacity. The numbers of androgen receptors vary among different ethnic groups. There may be little evidence of androgen excess despite high serum levels in individuals with few or no skin androgen receptors.

Many women don't know that it's abnormal to have dark hair growth on their bodies (especially face or low abdomen), and their healthcare providers may not notice dark hair if it has been waxed off or shaved. It's important to report dark hair growth to your healthcare provider because it can be a sign of PCOS.

Similarly, biochemical androgen excess includes elevated serum levels of androgens such as testosterone. Birth control pills will affect hormones levels, so they should not be checked until you have been off birth control for at least 4-6 weeks.

Ultrasound

A transvaginal ultrasound is an important diagnostic tool for PCOS. Polycystic ovaries on ultrasound are only present in about 75 percent of women with PCOS. The finding of 12 or more small follicles, in either ovary, meets the diagnostic criteria for polycystic ovaries (see Figure 2.1.). The follicles, usually located along the edge of the ovary, are often described as "a string of pearls." Follicular development stops prematurely so the follicles are usually between 4 to 8 millimeters in size. PCOS ovaries are typically enlarged; sometimes they are up to three times the normal size, which can lead to pelvic pain.

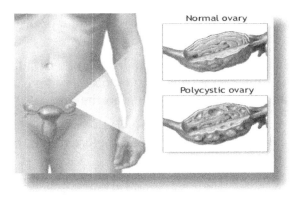

Figure 2.1. Normal versus polycystic ovary

Laboratory Tests

There is no consensus about which laboratory tests should be performed to diagnose PCOS. Tests may confirm PCOS and rule out other problems that may cause similar symptoms. Commonly the baseline tests include a TSH, total testosterone, DHEA-S, fasting glucose, fasting blood insulin, 17OH progesterone, and prolactin. Let's look at the rationale for each test:

- ❖ **TSH**: Thyroid problems can cause cycle irregularities and contribute to infertility. Testing the thyroid will rule out thyroid related causes for irregular cycles. Hypothyroidism (low thyroid) is a common problem and more common among women with PCOS.

- ❖ **Total Testosterone:** It should be less than 50 in women. Elevated testosterone (or clinical symptoms of androgen excess such as dark hair growth) meets one of the two diagnostic criteria for PCOS.

- ❖ **DHEA-S:** This is an androgen that is converted to testosterone. Elevated levels can be due to adrenal problems that can mimic PCOS. Slight elevations can be seen in PCOS.

- ❖ **Fasting blood glucose:** This helps screen for impaired fasting glucose (pre-diabetes) or diabetes. The impaired fasting glucose range is from 100 to 126. The diagnosis of diabetes is made with two or more fasting glucose levels over 126.

- ❖ **Fasting insulin:** This is used to screen for insulin resistance. The fasting insulin should be less than 10. To calculate a glucose-to-insulin ratio, divide the fasting glucose by the fasting insulin; a value of 4.5 or less may be suggestive of insulin resistance (for example a blood glucose of 80 divided by a fasting insulin of 20 = 4). Insulin levels may be helpful but are not always reliable and not necessary for diagnosing insulin resistance.

- ❖ **17OHProgesterone:** This test helps to rule out congenital adrenal hyperplasia (CAH) as CAH symptoms can mimic PCOS symptoms. The levels can also be elevated during pregnancy and while using fertility medication such as Clomid.

Prolonged anovulatory cycles can also cause an elevated level of 17OHprogesterone. If elevated, an ACTH Stimulation test can be done to confirm CAH.

❖ **Prolactin:** These levels can be elevated if there are pituitary problems such as a pituitary tumor. The test is done to rule out pituitary problems that can cause irregular cycles, which could mimic PCOS.

Other lab tests that are commonly ordered include FSH, LH, estradiol, progesterone, free testosterone, SHBG, CBC, HbA1c, oral glucose tolerance test, lipids, VAP, HsCRP, Free T3, Free T4, Vitamin B12 and Vitamin D depending on the person's symptoms and family history.

Women with PCOS should be screened for diabetes before the age of 30 due to the risk of early onset type 2 diabetes.

Chapter 3: Role of Insulin Resistance and Elevated Androgens

The two main problems in PCOS are insulin resistance and elevated androgens (mainly testosterone). With PCOS the ovaries are more sensitive to insulin. Elevated insulin levels stimulate the ovaries to produce androgens, which result in higher androgen levels. Androgen excess leads to anovulatory cycles and low progesterone, which contribute to irregular cycles. Elevated insulin levels also inhibit the production of sex hormone binding globulin by the liver, resulting in even more unbound or free androgens. It can become a vicious cycle.

Insulin resistance—seen in about 75 percent of women with PCOS—may be related to mutations in the insulin receptor gene that causes the insulin receptor to function abnormally and secrete higher than normal amounts of insulin. Don't think this is just a problem for people who have extra weight. Over-secretion of insulin is seen in both lean (normal weight) and obese women with PCOS.

According to the American Association of Clinical Endocrinologists it is prudent to regard all obese women and most nonobese women with PCOS as likely having insulin resistance and being at risk for insulin resistance syndrome (IRS). They also recommend consideration of Metformin therapy as the initial intervention for most women with PCOS.

Signs and Symptoms of Insulin Resistance

If you're resistant to insulin, then you may have these signs and symptoms:

- ❖ Craving sugar or simple carbohydrates
- ❖ Increased appetite
- ❖ Constant hunger
- ❖ Feeling shaky or irritable when hungry
- ❖ Fatigue after meals
- ❖ Inability to lose weight
- ❖ Physical aches and pains
- ❖ Central weight gain (mainly in the abdominal area)
- ❖ Acanthosis nigricans (dark skin)
- ❖ Skin tags
- ❖ Red bumps on upper arms (keratosis pilaris).

Acanthosis Nigricans

Insulin resistance can also cause a physical symptom called acanthosis nigricans, which is Latin for "black skin." In people with dark skin, it is easy to detect; it is dark soft skin on the back of the neck, elbows, underarms, upper-inner thighs, and across the knuckles. In lighter skinned people it can be more difficult to detect. The skin in those areas may appear to be tan or dirty, and the knees or elbows may be gray and rough. Insulin resistance from any cause can result in acanthosis nigricans.

How Insulin Resistance Develops

Today most calories in an average diet come in the form of carbohydrates, and most of those are simple carbohydrates (such as sugar, white flour, processed and fast foods) that quickly enter the bloodstream. The body has to release high levels of insulin to keep the level of glucose in the bloodstream from building up. Insulin resistance can stimulate the appetite and cause carbohydrate cravings because the cells are starved of glucose.

With prolonged levels of high insulin (hyperinsulinemia), the muscle, fat, and liver cells quit responding to this signal and the body becomes insulin resistant. Immediately, the body must release even more insulin to keep the blood sugar from getting too high. Hyperinsulinemia causes weight gain and then weight gain causes insulin resistance, so it becomes a vicious cycle and can result in rapid weight gain (see Figure 3.1.).

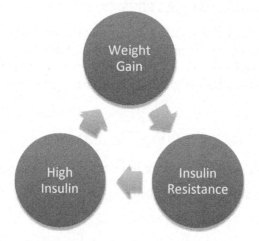

Figure 3.1. Vicious cycle of insulin resistance and weight gain

Seven Ways to Treat Insulin Resistance

1. **Moderate physical activity 3 to 5 times a week for at least 30 minutes.** Exercise encourages the body to transport blood sugar into the muscles as opposed to storing it as fat. In anticipation of this process, the body up-regulates its ability to utilize insulin, increasing sensitivity.

2. **Healthy diet.** A diet that consists primarily of lean meats and dairy; high-fiber grains, vegetables and legumes; leafy greens; and fruit will substantially aid the body's ability to balance insulin levels. Pairing complex carbs and protein also helps decrease the spike in glucose and insulin.

3. **Getting a good night's sleep.** Deep, restorative sleep—also called slow-wave sleep—helps regulate blood sugar. Getting adequate slow-wave sleep requires sleeping at least 6 to 7 hours per night, and it results in waking up feeling refreshed.

4. **Managing stress.** Stress results in the overproduction of cortisol, a hormone that counteracts the effect of insulin.

5. **Weight loss.** Weight loss can make the body more sensitive to insulin and lower blood glucose levels. Maintaining a lower body weight by eating fewer calories will also result in less demand for insulin.

6. **Medication.** Medication such as Metformin decreases insulin resistance and improves insulin sensitivity thereby helping the insulin the body makes work more effectively.

7. **Supplements.** Vitamins, dietary and herbal supplements such as inositol, magnesium, manganese, B vitamins, cinnamon, and chromium may also help with insulin resistance by increasing sensitivity.

Insulin Resistance Syndrome (AKA Metabolic Syndrome)

Insulin Resistance Syndrome (IRS) is a term championed by The American Association of Clinical Endocrinologists (AACE) to describe the consequences of insulin resistance and the compensating effects of high insulin. As mentioned previously, according to AACE it is prudent to regard all obese women and most nonobese women with PCOS as likely having insulin resistance and being at risk for insulin resistance syndrome (IRS).

Although insulin resistant individuals may secrete enough insulin to remain non-diabetic, they still have many of the same risk factors that people with diabetes have for long-term health complications. Screening for and treating IRS can decrease the risk for type 2 diabetes and cardiovascular disease.

According to an AACE position statement, the following are factors that increase the likelihood of IRS:

❖ Diagnosis of acanthosis nigricans, heart disease, high blood pressure, PCOS, or non-alcoholic or fatty liver disease (NAFLD)

❖ Family history of type 2 diabetes, high blood pressure or heart disease

❖ History of gestational diabetes or glucose intolerance

❖ Ethnicity other than Caucasian

❖ Sedentary lifestyle

❖ Body mass index over 25 (or waist circumference over 35 inches in women or 40 inches in men)

❖ Over 40 years of age.

The diagnosis of IRS requires at least 3 of these 5 criteria:

1. Triglycerides over 150

2. HDL cholesterol less than 40 in men or 50 in women

3. Blood pressure over 130/85

4. Fasting glucose 110-125 or 2 hour post glucose challenge 140-200

5. Central obesity (waist to hip ratio greater than 1.0).

Waist-to-Hip Ratio

People with waist-to-hip ratios (waist circumference divided by hip circumference) greater than 1.0 are considered *at risk* for insulin resistance. Higher waist-to-hip ratios indicate a greater proportion of weight is carried as abdominal fat. An ideal waist-to-hip ratio for women is less than 0.8.

Chapter 4: Treating PCOS

AACE Treatment Guidelines

In treatment, healthcare providers should focus on the following:

1. Recognizing the syndrome early.

2. Encouraging lifestyle modification, emphasizing controlled eating patterns and regular exercise.

3. Screening for diabetes and insulin resistance.

4. Managing lipid abnormalities with dietary modification, weight loss and/or medications as necessary.

5. Treating high blood pressure.

6. Measuring atherogenic markers such as CRP (for risk of heart disease).

7. Consideration of Metformin therapy as initial intervention in most women with PCOS.

8. Using an oral contraceptive pill or anti-androgens for skin problems associated with PCOS.

9. Using thiazolidinediones (TZDs) in patients with impaired glucose tolerance (pre-diabetes) or diabetes.

Additionally, I recommend treatment to include:

❖ Monitoring and remedying common vitamin deficiencies associated with PCOS, such as vitamin B12 and vitamin D deficiency. Vitamin B12 should always be added to Metformin therapy.

❖ Correcting hormone imbalances to protect against cancer of the uterus and for the physical and emotional benefits of hormone balancing.

Although there are a lot of intricacies to PCOS, try to avoid over complicating it. Develop treatment goals with your healthcare provider around the basics (such as correcting hormone imbalances and treating insulin resistance) and go from there.

An important variable when looking at treatment options is whether or not you are trying to conceive. See the following table (Figure 4.1.)

	Irregular Cycles	Low Progesterone	High Androgens	Insulin Resistance	Obesity
Trying to Conceive	Cycle with progesterone, progesterone challenge, weight loss	Progesterone supplementation	Treating insulin resistance will decrease androgens	Metformin, inositol, diet, exercise, weight loss	Metformin, inositol, diet, exercise
Not Trying to Conceive	OCPs, cycle with progesterone, progesterone challenge, weight loss	OCPs, progesterone supplementation	OCPs, Spironolactone, treating insulin resistance	Metformin, inositol, diet, exercise, weight loss	Metformin, inositol, diet, exercise, appetite suppressant

Figure 4.1. Treatment options for people trying to conceive and not trying to conceive.

Keep in mind that PCOS is a chronic condition and it's okay to take it one step at a time. Start with treating the most important or most distressing symptoms. Master one treatment goal or start one medication at a time, if necessary.

Build a relationship with your healthcare provider and follow up frequently to evaluate your progress with your treatment goals. It helps to be accountable to someone. For example, you are more likely to stick to your exercise and diet plan if you know you are going to be weighed regularly. Let your healthcare provider know that you need their support, knowledge, and expertise to help you proactively manage your condition and live a healthier life.

Medications

Metformin

Metformin is used to treat insulin resistance in type 2 diabetes and PCOS and it has well documented benefits. Metformin increases insulin sensitivity and inhibits glucose production from the liver without the risk of causing low blood sugar.

If you haven't tolerated Metformin in the past (typically due to GI side effects), then consider a sustained release tablet, increase the dose slowly, and decrease or eliminate simple sugars from your diet and you will tolerate it much better. The many benefits of Metformin include weight loss, reduction in carbohydrate cravings, cycle regulation, improved fertility, treating insulin resistance, lowering testosterone (improved acne, dark hair growth, and so on), and decreasing the risk for type 2 diabetes. It is also better tolerated when taken with a full meal. It is not unusual to see the shell of the sustained release tablet in bowel movements.

All people on Metformin should supplement with vitamin B12 (or be screened regularly for B12 deficiency). Vitamin B12 levels tend to be lower in women with PCOS and Metformin can further lower the levels. Vitamin B12 should be administered in the form of an injection, sublingual, or orally disintegrating tablet. Oral B12 may be less effective in treating B12 deficiency.

Actos and Avandia

Thiazolidenediones (TZDs), such as Actos and Avandia, are used to treat insulin resistance by increasing the efficiency of insulin receptors. TZDs can be used in combination with Metformin.

Januvia and Trajenta

DPP-4 inhibitors/Incretin Enhancers, such as Januvia and Trajenta, lower the glucose in response to a meal and reestablish first phase insulin release. They can be used in combination with Metformin.

Progesterone

Progesterone levels can be low due to anovulatory cycles. Low progesterone and estrogen predominance can lead to bleeding irregularities and increase the risk of pre-cancer and cancer of the uterus. Low progesterone can also increase the risk for miscarriage and preterm birth. Furthermore, chronic hormonal imbalances can also lead to PMS and depression. Cycling with progesterone (typically on cycle days 12 to 25) can help regulate cycles without preventing pregnancy. Women with low progesterone levels should supplement with progesterone when they become pregnant and continue taking it through the first trimester (or as directed by their healthcare provider) to decrease the risk of miscarriage.

Anti-Androgens

Anti-androgens, such as Spironolactone, are commonly used to lower testosterone and the effects of androgen excess such as acne, dark hair growth, and hair loss. It can take 3 to 6 months to see improvement in acne and 6 to 12 months to see improvement in dark hair growth and hair loss. Spironolactone can cause cycle irregularities if not used in combination with an OCP. It's also a pregnancy category D medication, so it's important to prevent pregnancy while taking it.

OCP/Hormone Birth Control

Hormone birth control can be used to regulate cycles, treat acne, and suppress dark hair growth by increasing sex hormone binding globulin (SHBG) and reducing lutenizing hormone (LH).

Appetite Suppressants

Appetite suppressants, such as phentermine, can help with weight loss. I have found the use of diet, exercise, Metformin, and appetite suppressants to be a successful combination for many of my PCOS patients. Frequently women with PCOS have struggled with weight gain despite their best efforts to be healthy, and they lose hope and motivation when their efforts fail to produce results.

Appetite suppressants are only used short-term, but the increased energy and appetite suppression can help with motivation and self control while healthier eating and exercise patterns are established.

Supplements

Vitamins, dietary, and herbal supplements such as inositol, magnanese, B vitamins, cinnamon, and chromium may also help with insulin resistance by increasing sensitivity.

Diet/Lifestyle Change

Many opinions and schools of thought exist on the diet that individuals with PCOS should follow, varying from low to moderate carbohydrate diets. Some recommend excluding grains altogether while some just recommend excluding gluten containing grains, and so on. After much reading and research, I decided to put my trust in the research and expertise of a PCOS Expert and Registered Dietician Angela Grassi, RD.

She recommends **pairing** approximately 30 to 45 grams of complex carbohydrates per meal and 15 grams of complex carbohydrates per snack with lean protein. She also recommends cutting out (or at least drastically decreasing) the intake of processed foods and simple sugars.

Meals should consist of approximately 50 percent complex carbohydrates, 30 percent lean protein, and 20 percent healthy fats. Pairing complex carbohydrates with protein decreases the rate at which carbohydrates are turned to sugar in your bloodstream. Avoiding spikes in blood sugar levels helps to avoid spikes in insulin levels.

If an individual feels better or has more success with weight loss following a low carbohydrate diet, then I would certainly support that, but I think it's important to make changes that can be sustained over time. "Dieting" does not work, at least not long-term. If you change the way you eat to lose weight and then go back to eating your normal diet, then you will gain the weight back. That's just common sense, right? So *why* are we so surprised when it happens?

The key to losing weight (and maintaining it) is being consistent over time. It can get discouraging when you're working hard and the weight loss is slow. After a week maybe you've only lost a pound, but what does losing a pound a week look like in 20 weeks, 30 weeks or 50 weeks? How would you like to be 52 pounds lighter a year from now?

I strongly recommend a referral to a Registered Dietician (RD) for dietary counseling and individualized meal planning. Remember, this is not a diet but a lifestyle change.

It is ideal to see an RD who is experienced with PCOS or a diabetic educator. If you live in an area where an RD is unavailable or you are unable to find an RD with experience in PCOS, then I recommend a dietary consultation (by Skype) with Angela Grassi, RD, or one of her associates. Please contact them at PCOSnutrition.com.

You can also order her book *The PCOS Workbook* by Angela Grassi, RD, and Stephanie Mattei, Psy.D. They also offer a PCOS Cookbook.

Exercise/Weight Loss

As noted before, moderate physical activity 3 to 5 times a week for at least 30 minutes also helps reduce insulin resistance. Also, exercise helps emotionally as well as physically. The endorphins released during exercise can help combat anxiety and depression too.

Weight loss lowers testosterone, LH, blood glucose, and insulin, and it improves the lipid profile and can restore normal ovulation. An improvement in dark hair growth is also seen from lowered testosterone levels and increased SHBG, resulting in less unbound or free testosterone.

Chapter 5: Infertility

Infertility, a painful and devastating disease, is a common condition affecting about 15 percent of couples. The emotional pain and suffering associated with infertility has been compared to the pain and suffering of those diagnosed with cancer. Yet half of infertile couples fail to seek treatment and suffer in silence. While some women with PCOS are infertile, most women with PCOS ovulate intermittently. Conception may take longer than in other women, or women with PCOS may have fewer children than they had planned due to the prolonged period between ovulatory cycles.

Infertility is defined as the inability to conceive after one year for women 35 and under or the inability to conceive within 6 months for women over 35. The reason for infertility is approximately 40 percent female factor, 40 percent male factor, and 20 percent unexplained.

Anovulation (not ovulating) is the most common reason for female factor infertility, and PCOS is the most common reason for anovulation. It can be corrected through weight reduction (as little as 10 percent weight reduction can restore ovulation for many women), Metformin, and medications that stimulate ovulation such as Clomid.

Many women with PCOS first seek treatment for fertility from their OB/GYN or women's health practitioner. If a woman is over 35 or does not conceive within six months while using Metformin and/or Clomid, then she should be offered a referral to a Reproductive Endocrinologist. Women who are not ovulating consistently should be worked up for PCOS.

Note: Treating a person with Clomid without a proper work-up has much the same effect as prescribing birth control for irregular cycles without a proper work-up. It may result in delaying the diagnosis and incomplete treatment, and it may create a missed opportunity to diagnose PCOS and allow the person to get proper treatment. Remember, understanding your diagnosis and getting proper treatment will not only improve your chances of getting pregnant, but also it will improve your overall health now and in the future.

While facilitating a PCOS support group, I discovered that most women who deal with infertility experience emotional pain. They feel bad that they can't have children. They report feeling jealous of friends and family members who are expecting babies. Some women have a hard time participating in baby-focused events such as baby showers, baby blessings, christenings, and so on. Their jealousy then leads to guilt or shame.

They also report feeling alone and isolated. As well, they say that initially everyone has advice (that is usually more embarrassing than helpful), but eventually the subject becomes taboo and no one talks about it.

Many couples fail to seek treatment for infertility because they think it is too expensive and the only option is in vitro fertilization (IVF). The truth is, the majority of couples can succeed in becoming pregnant with minimal expense and treatment and only about 10 percent of couples will require IVF to conceive.

When you become pregnant, it is important to know that women with PCOS can have a higher rate of pregnancy complications (including miscarriage, gestational diabetes, preeclampsia, and preterm birth) compared to women without PCOS. Your healthcare provider may recommend progesterone supplementation, Metformin, and more frequent appointments during your pregnancy. Ask your healthcare provider about the signs of preterm labor and other things you can do to improve your chances of a healthy, full-term pregnancy.

Chapter 6: Psychological Aspects of PCOS

Being diagnosed with a chronic illness can be devastating especially when it can affect a person's physical appearance, ability to conceive, hormone balance, and general health. Women with PCOS often struggle with weight gain, dark hair growth, and acne, which can lead to problems with body image, depression, and anxiety.

Hormonal imbalances can increase the risk for PMS, depression, anxiety, and eating disorders. Infertility can lead to anxiety, hopelessness, isolation, and depression. For these, and other reasons, psychological counseling may be beneficial.

Eating Disorders and Altered Body Image

Eating disorders and body image issues can be problematic for women with PCOS. Many factors affect body image and contribute to the development of eating disorders such as anorexia nervosa, bulimia nervosa, and binge-eating disorder.

Why does one develop an eating disorder? Eating disorders develop more to feel in control than to eat. Food helps the person feel in control and avoid painful feelings. Cultural ideals, family attitudes, emotional disorders, metabolic disorders, stressful events, and even normal dieting can lead to altered body images and eating disorders.

In the US, thinness is a social ideal and some people define themselves by how physically attractive they are. Magazines create an unrealistic body image for the average woman to attain.

Attitudes about weight can be established in early childhood by the attitudes of parents and family members. Emotional disorders such as depression and anxiety can contribute to emotional eating.

Metabolic problems such as insulin resistance can cause carbohydrate cravings that lead to binge eating. Stressful life situations are also a cause, such as starting a new job, relocating, getting married, or divorced, or trauma such as sexual assault.

Even normal dieting can be a problem. Losing weight can feel good and bring positive attention, but it can be taken to an extreme. Getting the right help is important to recover from an eating disorder. Ask your healthcare provider to refer you to a counselor who specialized in eating disorders or an eating disorder support group, for best results.

Psychology of Change/Forming New Habits

Being diagnosed with PCOS can be overwhelming and you may be asked to make a lot of changes to your lifestyle to become healthier and reduce your symptoms of PCOS.

Making real changes and seeing real results take consistent effort. We've all struggled with changing habits especially if we try to make too many changes at once (that's why New Year's resolutions fail so often).

I was motivated to learn more about the psychology of change after seeing many of my patients struggle to maintain change even when they were feeling better and seeing amazing results by eating healthier, exercising, taking their medications, and so on.

I found a website called zenhabits.net. The author, Leo Babauta, talks a lot about changing habits and had a blog post entitled "The Habit Change Cheat Sheet: 29 Ways to Successfully Ingrain a Behavior" (see Appendix C).

The habit change information made a lot of sense to me, so I started sharing it with my patients, and they have loved it! Babauta encourages his non-copyrighted work to be shared because he understands the value of helping people replace bad habits with healthy habits. An overweight smoker with a lot of debt, he transformed himself into a healthy, debt-free and smoke-free person who runs marathons.

Chapter 7: PCOS Education

FAQ Handout

PCOS patient education is important and fortunately there is a lot of information available. The U.S. Department of Health and Human Services, Office on Women's Services has a great handout entitled *Polycystic Ovary Syndrome (PCOS) Frequently Asked Questions*(see Appendix D). The handout is free of copyright so it can be reproduced and shared. It is six pages long and answers 12 common questions about PCOS, including:

1. What is polycystic ovary syndrome?
2. How many women have PCOS?
3. What causes PCOS?
4. What are the symptoms of PCOS?
5. Why do women with PCOS have trouble with their menstrual cycle and fertility?
6. Does PCOS change at menopause?
7. How do I know if I have PCOS?
8. How is PCOS treated?
9. How does PCOS affect a woman while pregnant?
10. Does PCOS put women at risk for other health problems?
11. I have PCOS what can I do to prevent complications?
12. How can I cope with the emotional effects of PCOS?

PCOS Basics Handout

I have also included a copy of a handout I call the *PCOS Basics Handout* (see Appendix E). I created this one-page handout because I was constantly writing sticky notes with recommended supplements or the titles of recommended readings and so on. It offers a brief explanation of PCOS, the goals of treatment, an explanation of the PCOS diet, the benefits of seeing a dietician for dietary counseling, the reasons for seeing a counselor for psychological counseling, the benefits of exercise, a list of vitamins and supplements, the name and website of a PCOS book I recommend, and information on the PCOS support group offered in our clinic.

Nutritional Handouts

I give nutritional handouts to my patients that I ordered from PCOSnutrition.com (PCOS Food Exchanges, Mindful Eating Exercises, How Food Affects Insulin Levels, Four Sample Meal Plans, etc.). I find these especially helpful for patients who are unable to see a dietician because of the expense. Sometimes they do not have insurance and other times their insurance will not pay for dietary counseling for PCOS. I have found that some insurance companies will pay for dietary counseling if the patient has impaired glucose, obesity or dyslipidemia (high cholesterol or triglycerides).

Chapter 8: Multidisciplinary Approach to Care

Managing every aspect of PCOS is important to improve your quality of life and reduce the risk of long-term health problems. The symptoms of PCOS overlap several areas of medicine. Here's a list of specialists who may be involved in your care with an explanation of their expertise as it relates to treating PCOS. Don't hesitate to ask for a referral.

- ❖ **Primary Care Provider/PCP** (Family Practice Physician, Internist, CNM, Nurse Practitioner or PA): Many women with PCOS present to their primary care provider with complaints such as irregular cycles, weight gain, acne, fatigue, anxiety, depression, eating disorders, and difficulty getting pregnant. A primary care provider can work up and treat the condition and make referrals, as necessary, so the patient can receive comprehensive care for PCOS.

- ❖ **OB/GYN:** An OB/GYN specializes in women's health, including reproductive health, pregnancy, labor, and delivery. Many women with PCOS present to an OB/GYN with complaints of irregular cycles, weight gain, acne, fatigue, difficulty getting pregnant, and/or recurrent miscarriage. An OB/GYN can act as a primary care provider and make referrals as necessary to provide the comprehensive care the patient with PCOS needs.

- ❖ **Registered Dietician (RD):** A Registered Dietician can teach people about nutrition, a PCOS diet, and meal planning. Ask for a referral to an RD who has experience working with PCOS, if possible, or at least experience working with diabetic patients. It is so important for women to understand the role of nutrition in treating insulin resistance since insulin resistance is a core problem in PCOS.

- ❖ **Psychologist/Therapist/Support Group:** Psychological counseling should be considered by people with PCOS who are struggling emotionally. Being diagnosed with a chronic illness can be devastating, especially when it can affect an individual's physical appearance, ability to conceive, hormone balance, and general health. Patients with PCOS can struggle with anxiety, body image problems, depression, eating disorders, hormonal imbalances, infertility, and PMS.

- ❖ **Reproductive Endocrinologist:** A Reproductive Endocrinologist is an OB/GYN with advanced education and training in male and female reproduction and infertility. They can diagnose and manage PCOS. Their primary focus tends to be infertility management, and they may manage PCOS long-term or have a patient's PCP, OB/GYN, or endocrinologist manage PCOS long-term.

- ❖ **Endocrinologist:** Endocrinologists specialize in hormonal conditions such as pituitary, adrenal and thyroid disorders, diabetes, and PCOS. Depending on their practice they may manage PCOS or serve as a consultant to your PCP or OB/GYN.

- ❖ **Internist:** Internists are physicians who specialize in preventing, diagnosing, and treating chronic conditions such as hypertension, hyperlipidemia, and diabetes. They may consult with your PCP or OB/GYN or serve as your PCP.

- ❖ **Dermatologist:** Dermatologists specialize in diagnosing and treating conditions related to the skin and hair. They can help you treat problems with acne, excessive dark hair growth (on the face and body), and male pattern hair loss.

Chapter 9: PCOS Support Group and Success Stories

Support Group

The idea for a PCOS support group came to me while I was visiting with a PCOS patient. She expressed how alone she felt in her illness. She happened to be the fourth PCOS patient I had seen that day, so I decided I needed to do something to bring these women together. I realized there are so many women dealing with these same issues, yet they all feel isolated.

We sponsored a PCOS Awareness booth at a local women's expo and asked people to sign up if they were interested in a local PCOS support group. In the end, we had about 50 women sign up—quite a large number. Then we sent out an email to our active PCOS patients asking about interest in a local support group and got a positive response too, so we started a support group.

We have had speakers from different specialties come and talk about PCOS issues related to their area of expertise. We have had a Registered Dietician talk about PCOS diet, a Therapist talk about eating disorders, a Reproductive Endocrinologist discuss infertility, a Chaplain talk about the grief and loss associated with chronic medical conditions, and a Dermatologist talk about acne and hirsutism.

We do a free raffle for prizes and serve healthy refreshments. We ask for donations (suggested $3/person) to cover expenses. We also started a blog and a Facebook page.

Maybe you can join or start a support group in your area!

Success Stories

Through the proactive management of PCOS, I have seen so many women transform their lives and accomplish things they had given up hope of achieving. It's amazing to witness the changes that balancing hormones, treating insulin resistance, and losing weight can bring: having more energy, feeling better emotionally, feeling beautiful, running a marathon, getting pregnant, and so on. I hope that sharing some success stories* will inspire you to proactively treat PCOS. You are the author of your own story! Why not make it a success story?

Success Story #1

Kate was 29 years old, she had been diagnosed with PCOS as a teenager. She started putting on weight rapidly, going from 210 to 270 pounds over 3 years. She disliked the amount of dark facial hair she had developed and felt fatigued and out of balance hormonally. She had tried to conceive for 8 years but had given up. She decided it was time to lose weight and get her health back on track so she could feel better. She started Metformin, Spironolactone, Vitamin B12, Vitamin D3, and a multiple vitamin. She met with a dietician and modified her diet, cutting out soda, limiting simple sugars, eating more whole foods, and pairing complex carbs with protein. She also started exercising at a local cross training gym with some of her coworkers. After a few months, she was a little discouraged with her slow progress so we added an appetite suppressant that helped augment her weight loss. She reported more energy, decreased appetite, and fewer carb cravings, and she lost 50 pounds over 6 months. Her goal was to lose weight to feel better and decrease her PCOS symptoms. In addition to meeting those goals, she also got pregnant with her "miracle baby" as she calls her.

Success story #2

Allie was 18 years old with newly diagnosed PCOS and binge eating disorder. She had put on so much weight over the course of a year that she stopped hanging out with friends or socializing much because she felt embarrassed by her size. She came in asking for help with weight loss. She was excited to learn more about PCOS and readily accepted a referral to see a dietician and a counselor who specializes in eating disorders. Between a healthy diet, exercise, medication, and counseling she lost 60 pounds over the following 8 months. When she came in for a follow up appointment, she said something that really touched my heart: She told me that she recently passed a mirror and caught a glimpse of herself and felt beautiful for the first time in years. She understands the way she feels about herself is a result of the emotional as well as physical transformation she has experienced.

Success Story #3

Diagnosed with PCOS at age 19, Melissa didn't take the diagnosis seriously and failed to keep her follow-up appointment. From age 19 to 24 she gained 75 pounds. She was 24 when she got married and tried to conceive for a year without success. She was embarrassed to come back and see me. As a result, she sought treatment from another provider and was started on Clomid, which she took for six months without success. She decided to take a break from trying to get pregnant to lose some weight and get healthier. In the end, however, she felt like I was the person who could help her achieve her goals so she finally followed up with me. She was motivated. Between a healthy eating plan, daily walking, and medication (Metformin and progesterone), she lost 50 pounds in 6 months and conceived without fertility medication.

Success Story #4

Jade was 28 years old with newly diagnosed PCOS. She was a runner with several marathons under her belt. She always felt like she was "thicker and bigger boned" than anyone else in her family. She stated she had to exercise every day and practically starve herself to maintain her weight. She did well when she was started on OCPs and Metformin. They allowed her to eat a wider variety of whole foods (such as fruit and whole grains that she has previously avoided) and still lose weight. The changes she made helped her successfully lose 15 pounds over 4 months, decrease a pant size, and cut 23 minutes off her marathon time.

Success Story #5

Monica was 35 years old with known PCOS. She was going through a divorce and had gained a lot of weight, felt depressed and exhausted, had a short temper and was getting in trouble at work for performance and attitude issues. She felt like she had hit rock bottom and decided it was time to seek treatment for PCOS and depression. She started taking a rigorous karate class 3 nights a week and cutting out soda and simple sugars from her diet. She also started medication (Metformin, progesterone, and Prozac), vitamins, and supplements. She also started psychotherapy with a counselor. Over the following 6 months she lost 40 pounds, balanced her moods, and "got her groove back," as she puts it.

Success Story #6

Carrie was 40 years old with known PCOS. She had been told she was pre-diabetic and decided to take charge of her health to avoid ending up with type 2 diabetes like both of her parents. On her initial lab work her inflammatory markers (that evaluate for cardiovascular risk) were so high that we thought there had been a lab error and immediately repeated them. Unfortunately, the numbers were correct. She met with a dietician and started a healthy eating plan, exercise, and medication (Metformin, B/P med, cholesterol lowering med, vitamins and supplements). She struggled with giving up her favorite candy, but eventually she did, and over the course of a year she lost 40 pounds. In addition to losing weight and feeling much better, she remains non-diabetic and her inflammatory markers are completely normal.

Success Story #7

Sharon was 21 years old with newly diagnosed PCOS. A beautiful girl, she would not get within 10 feet of another person because she was so self conscious of the dark hair on her face. She had aunts with terrible facial hair problems and had been told if she shaved or plucked the hair it would get worse. She had spent years feeling hopeless and ugly and had isolated herself as a result. Treating her PCOS with diet, birth control pills, Spironolactone, and Vaniqa changed this young woman's life. She found love and got engaged within a year of starting treatment for PCOS.

Success Story #8

Jodi was 25 years old with newly diagnosed PCOS. She had a sister with PCOS and started seeing symptoms in herself, such as irregular cycles and dark hair growth. She was very thin and had type 1 diabetes. She felt bothered by the PCOS symptoms but her biggest complaint was marked fatigue for the past three years. She had previously had testing for hypothyroidism, anemia, vitamin deficiencies, mono, chronic fatigue and all of the typical tests that would be done for fatigue but nothing showed up. The fatigue was so debilitating that she had to take several naps a day, and she and her husband had delayed having children because she did not feel she could be a good mother due to her health.

Her work-up revealed PCOS with insulin resistance. So the insulin she injected was not working efficiently, and she was having a hard time controlling her blood sugars. She started Metformin and within the first month she reported the fatigue was gone. She came in for her follow-up appointment and hugged me and told me she felt like she had her life back. Over time she has significantly decreased her insulin dose to about a 1/3 of what she was using before she started treating insulin resistance with diet, exercise, and Metformin.

*Names and some details have been changed to protect privacy.

Chapter 10: PCOS Resources, Blogs and Online Support

Resources

A number of organizations deal with the many physical and psychological problems I've described. They can help you get more information on treatments and practitioners.

- ❖ American Association of Clinical Endocrinologists (www.aace.com)
- ❖ American College of OB/GYN (www.acog.org)
- ❖ American Diabetes Association (www.diabetes.org)
- ❖ American Heart Association (www.americanheart.org)
- ❖ American Psychological Association (www.apa.org)
- ❖ American Society for Reproductive Medicine (www.asrm.org)
- ❖ National Eating Disorders Association (www.edap.org)
- ❖ OBGYN.net (www.obgyn.net)
- ❖ RESOLVE The National Infertility Association (www.resolve.org)

Apps and Online Support

In this digital age, there's an app for everything, right? Consider using one of the following fitness apps to help with your treatment:

- ❖ iperiod
- ❖ loseit
- ❖ mapmywalk
- ❖ myfitnesspal
- ❖ runningit
- ❖ wahoofitness

The web provides numerous places where you can discuss PCOS and learn from others with the condition:

- ❖ PCOS Nutrition (www.PCOSnutrition.com)
- ❖ PCOS Pals (www.health.groups.yahoo.com/group/PCOS-Pals/)
- ❖ PCOS Today Magazine (www.PCOStodaymagazine.com)
- ❖ PCOS UK (www.pcos-uk.org.uk)
- ❖ Polycystic Ovary Syndrome of Australia (www.posaa.asn.au)
- ❖ Project PCOS (www.projectPCOS.org)
- ❖ Soulcysters (www.soulcysters.com)
- ❖ Thriving with PCOS (thrivingwithPCOS.com)

Appendix A: Glossary of terms

1. Amenorrhea: The absence of a menstrual period for three months in a woman of reproductive age.

2. Androgens: Hormones that control the development and maintenance of male sex characteristics. Androgens include testosterone, dihydrotestosterone and androstenedione. A subset of androgens, adrenal androgens, includes DHEA, DHEA-S and dehydroepiandrosterone.

3. Androgen excess: A medical condition characterized by excessive production and/or secretion of androgens.

4. Anovulation/anovulatory cycle: A menstrual cycle during which the ovaries do not release an oocyte. Therefore, ovulation does not take place.

5. Complex carbohydrates: Whole foods that have not been processed, such as whole grain breads, fruits, and vegetables.

6. Dysfunctional uterine bleeding (DUB): Abnormal bleeding or an irregular menstrual cycle due to a hormonal imbalance. About 90 percent of DUB occurs due to anovulatory menstrual cycles.

7. Dyslipidemia: Abnormal amounts of fats (like cholesterol and triglycerides) in the blood. This is often due to diet and lifestyle but can also be genetic. Prolonged elevation of insulin levels can also lead to dyslipidemia.

8. Follicles (ovarian): Round cells found in the ovary that contain a single oocyte (immature ovum or egg). They develop once a month in humans and culminate in ovulation.

9. Follicle stimulating hormone (FSH): A hormone synthesized and secreted by the anterior pituitary gland that regulates development, growth, pubertal maturation, and reproduction.

10. Healthcare provider: A health care professional within medicine, midwifery, nursing, pharmacy, or allied health professions.

11. Hirsutism: Excessive hair growth on women where terminal hair growth does not usually occur such as the face, chest, abdomen, and back.

12. Hyperinsulinemia: A condition in which there is an excess of insulin circulating in the blood relative to the level of glucose.

13. Hypoglycemia: Low blood sugar. A term also used for a common condition characterized by shakiness and altered mood and thinking treated by eating balanced meals and avoiding simple sugars.

14. Infertility: The inability to conceive after one year (women 35 and under) or after 6 months (women over 35).

15. Insulin: A peptide hormone produced by the pancreas that causes cells in skeletal muscles and fat cells to absorb glucose from the blood.

16. Insulin resistance: A physiologic condition in which cells fail to respond to the normal actions of insulin.

17. Lutenizing hormone (LH): A hormone produced in the anterior pituitary. In females, an acute raise or "surge" in LH triggers ovulation. Ovulation predictor tests detect LH.

18. Menorrhagia: Abnormally heavy and long menstrual period (lasting longer than 7 days) that occurs at regular intervals.

19. Oligomenorrhea: Irregular menstrual periods occurring at intervals of more than 35 days apart and resulting in 9 or fewer menstrual cycles per year.

20. Oligoovulation: Irregular or infrequent ovulation.

21. Sex hormone binding globulin (SHBG): A glycoprotein that binds to sex hormones such as androgens and estrogen.

22. Simple carbohydrates: The most basic units of carbohydrates and the simplest form of sugar (glucose, fructose and galactose). Also refer to foods that are processed or refined and turn to sugar quickly once they enter the blood stream.

23. Testosterone: A hormone that controls the development and maintenance of male sex characteristics. Often excreted in excess in PCOS.

Appendix B: Diagnostic Criteria

Three different diagnostic criteria are used for diagnosing PCOS. They are similar, but the Rotterdam Consensus is the only one that does not require androgen excess to be part of the diagnostic criteria. If a woman has irregular cycles and polycystic ovaries, and other causes have been ruled out, she has PCOS with or without signs of androgen excess.

1. **National Institute of Health (NIH)**

   In 1990, a consensus workshop sponsored by the NIH/NICHD suggested that a person has PCOS if she has all of the following:

   a. Oligoovulation or anovulation manifested by oligomenorrhea or amenorrhea

   b. Signs of androgen excess (clinical or biochemical)

   c. Other entities are excluded that could mimic symptoms of polycystic ovary syndrome.

2. **Rotterdam Consensus**

   At the Rotterdam revised consensus meeting sponsored by ESHRE/ASRM in 2003, it was proposed that at least two of the following three findings serve as the diagnostic criteria for PCOS:

   a. Oligoovulation on anovulation manifested by oligomenorrhea or amenorrhea

   b. Clinical or biochemical androgen excess

   c. Polycystic ovaries on pelvic ultrasound.

   It was also recommended to exclude other conditions that would cause androgen excess or mimic PCOS symptoms.

3. **Androgen Excess**

   In 2006, The Androgen Excess PCOS Society suggested the following diagnostic criteria for PCOS:

   a. Excess androgen activity

   b. Oligomenorrhea or amenorrhea and/or polycystic ovaries

   c. Other entities are excluded that would cause androgen excess.

Appendix C: The Habit Change Cheat Sheet

29 Ways to Successfully Ingrain a Behavior:

1. Do just one habit at a time. Extremely important. Habit change is difficult, even with just one habit. If you do more than one habit at a time, you're setting yourself up for failure.

2. Start small. The smaller the better, because habit change is difficult, and trying to take on too much is a recipe for disaster. Want to exercise? Start with just 5-10 minutes. Want to wake up earlier? Try just 10 minutes earlier for now.

3. Do a 30-day Challenge. In my experience, it takes about 30 days to change a habit, if you're focused and consistent.

4. Write it down. Just saying you're going to change the habit is not enough of a commitment. You need to actually write it down, on paper.

5. Make a plan. While you're writing, also write down a plan. This will ensure you're really prepared. The plan should include your reasons (motivations) for changing, obstacles, triggers, support buddies, and other ways you're going to make this a success. More on each of these below.

6. Know your motivations, and be sure they're strong. Write them down in your plan. You have to be very clear why you're doing this, and the benefits of doing it need to be clear in your head.

7. Don't start right away. In your plan, write down a start date. Maybe a week or two from the date you start writing out the plan. Make this a Big Day. It builds up anticipation and excitement, and helps you to prepare.

8. Write down all your obstacles. If you've tried this habit change before (odds are you have), you've likely failed. Reflect on those failures, and figure out what stopped you from succeeding. Write down every obstacle that's happened to you, and others that are likely to happen. Then write down how you plan to overcome them. That's the key: write down your solution before the obstacles arrive, so you're prepared.

9. Identify your triggers. What situations trigger your current habit? For a smoking habit, for example, triggers might include waking in the morning, having coffee, drinking alcohol, stressful meetings, going out with friends, driving, etc. Most habits have multiple triggers. Identify all of them and write them in your plan.

10. For every single trigger, identify a positive habit you're going to do instead. When you first wake in the morning, instead of smoking, what will you do? What about when you get stressed? When you go out with friends? Some positive habits could include: exercise, meditation, deep breathing, organizing, decluttering, and more.

11. Plan a support system. Who will you turn to when you have a strong urge? Write these people into your plan. Online support forums are a great tool as well. Don't underestimate the power of support—it's really important.

12. Ask for help. Get your family and friends and coworkers to support you. Ask them for their help, and let them know how important this is.

13. Become aware of self-talk. You talk to yourself, in your head, all the time—but often we're not aware of these thoughts. Start listening. Often they are negative: "I can't do this. This is too difficult. Why am I putting myself through this? I'm not strong enough." It's important to know you're doing this.

14. Stay positive. You will have negative thoughts—the important thing is to realize when you're having them, and push them out of your head. Squash them like a bug! Then replace them with a positive thought. "I can do this!"

15. Have strategies to defeat the urge. Urges come and go—they're inevitable, and they're strong. But they're also temporary, and beatable. Urges usually last about a minute or two, and they come in waves of varying strength. You just need to ride out the wave, and the urge will go away. Try deep breathing, take a walk, call a support buddy, etc.

16. Prepare for the sabotagers. There will always be people who are negative, who try to get you to do your old habit. Be ready for them. Confront them, and be direct: you don't need them to try to sabotage you, you need their support, and if they can't support you then you don't want to be around them.

17. Talk to yourself. Be your own cheerleader, give yourself pep talks, repeat your mantra (below) and don't be afraid to seem crazy to others. We'll see who's crazy when you've changed your habit and they're still lazy, unhealthy slobs!

18. Have a mantra. For quitting smoking, mine was: "Not One Puff Ever".

19. Use visualization. This is powerful. Vividly picture, in your head, successfully changing your habit. This seems new-agey, but it really works.

20. Have rewards. Regular ones. You might see these as bribes, but actually they are just positive feedback. Put these into your plan, along with the milestones at which you'll receive them.

21. Take it one urge at a time. Often we're told to take it one day at a time—which is good advice—but really it's one urge at a time. Just make it through this urge.

22. Not One Puff Ever (in other words, no exceptions). This seems harsh, but it's a necessity: when you're trying to break the bonds between an old habit and a trigger, and form a new bond between the trigger and a new habit, you need to be really consistent. So, at least for 30 days (and preferably 60), you need to have no exceptions. Each time a trigger happens, you need to do the new habit and not the old one.

23. Get rest. Being tired leaves us vulnerable to relapse. Get a lot of rest so you can have the energy to overcome the urges.

24. Drink lots of water. Similar to the item above, being dehydrated leaves us open to failure. Stay hydrated.

25. Renew your commitment often. Remind yourself of your commitment hourly, and at the beginning and end of each day.

26. Set up public accountability. Blog about it, post on a forum, email your commitment and daily progress to friends and family. When we make it public—not just the commitment but the progress updates—we don't want to fail.

27. Engineer it so it's hard to fail. Create a groove that's harder to get out of than to stay in: increase positive feedback for sticking with the habit, and increase negative feedback for not doing the habit.

28. Avoid some situations where you normally do your old habit, at least for awhile, to make it a bit easier on yourself. Realize, though, when you go back to those situations, you will still get the old urges, and when that happens you should be prepared.

29. If you fail, figure out what went wrong, plan for it, and try again. Don't let failure and guilt stop you. They're just obstacles, but they can be overcome.

Appendix D: U.S. Health and Human Services PCOS FAQ

http://www.womenshealth.gov

1-800-994-9662

TDD: 1-888-220-5446

Polycystic Ovary Syndrome (PCOS)

Q: What is polycystic ovary syndrome (PCOS)?

A: Polycystic (pah-lee-SIS-tik) ovary syndrome (PCOS) is a health problem that can affect a woman's:

- Menstrual cycle
- Ability to have children
- Hormones
- Heart
- Blood vessels
- Appearance

With PCOS, women typically have:

- High levels of androgens (AN-druh-junz). These are sometimes called male hormones, though females also make them.
- Missed or irregular periods (monthly bleeding)
- Many small cysts (sists) (fluid-filled sacs) in their ovaries

Q: How many women have PCOS?

A: Between 1 in 10 and 1 in 20 women of childbearing age has PCOS. As many as 5 million women in the United States may be affected. It can occur in girls as young as 11 years old.

Q: What causes PCOS?

A: The cause of PCOS is unknown. But most experts think that several factors, including genetics, could play a role. Women with PCOS are more likely to have a mother or sister with PCOS.

A main underlying problem with PCOS is a hormonal imbalance. In women with PCOS, the ovaries make more androgens than normal. Androgens are male hormones that females also make. High levels of these hormones affect the development and release of eggs during ovulation.

Researchers also think insulin may be linked to PCOS. Insulin is a hormone that controls the change of sugar, starches, and other food into energy for the body to use or store. Many women with PCOS have too much insulin in their bodies because they have problems using it. Excess insulin appears to increase production of androgen. High androgen levels can lead to:

- Acne
- Excessive hair growth
- Weight gain
- Problems with ovulation

Q: What are the symptoms of PCOS?

A: The symptoms of PCOS can vary from woman to woman. Some of the symptoms of PCOS include:

- Infertility (not able to get pregnant) because of not ovulating. In fact, PCOS is the most common cause of female infertility.
- Infrequent, absent, and/or irregular menstrual periods
- Hirsutism (HER-suh-tiz-um) — increased hair growth on the face, chest, stomach, back, thumbs, or toes

page 1

U.S. Department of Health and Human Services, Office on Women's Health

http://www.womenshealth.gov

1-800-994-9662

TDD: 1-888-220-5446

- Cysts on the ovaries
- Acne, oily skin, or dandruff
- Weight gain or obesity, usually with extra weight around the waist
- Male-pattern baldness or thinning hair
- Patches of skin on the neck, arms, breasts, or thighs that are thick and dark brown or black
- Skin tags — excess flaps of skin in the armpits or neck area
- Pelvic pain
- Anxiety or depression
- Sleep apnea — when breathing stops for short periods of time while asleep

Q: Why do women with PCOS have trouble with their menstrual cycle and fertility?

A: The ovaries, where a woman's eggs are produced, have tiny fluid-filled sacs called follicles or cysts. As the egg grows, the follicle builds up fluid. When the egg matures, the follicle breaks open, the egg is released, and the egg travels through the fallopian tube to the uterus (womb) for fertilization. This is called ovulation.

In women with PCOS, the ovary doesn't make all of the hormones it needs for an egg to fully mature. The follicles may start to grow and build up fluid but ovulation does not occur. Instead, some follicles may remain as cysts. For these reasons, ovulation does not occur and the hormone progesterone is not made. Without progesterone, a woman's menstrual cycle is irregular or absent. Plus, the ovaries make male hormones, which also prevent ovulation.

page 2

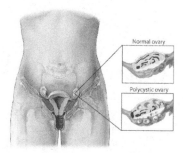

Normal ovary

Polycystic ovary

Q: Does PCOS change at menopause?

A: Yes and no. PCOS affects many systems in the body. So, many symptoms may persist even though ovarian function and hormone levels change as a woman nears menopause. For instance, excessive hair growth continues, and male-pattern baldness or thinning hair gets worse after menopause. Also, the risks of complications (health problems) from PCOS, such as heart attack, stroke, and diabetes, increase as a woman gets older.

Q: How do I know if I have PCOS?

A: There is no single test to diagnose PCOS. Your doctor will take the following steps to find out if you have PCOS or if something else is causing your symptoms.

Medical History. Your doctor will ask about your menstrual periods, weight changes, and other symptoms.

Physical Exam. Your doctor will want to measure your blood pressure, body mass index (BMI), and waist size. He or she also will check the areas of increased hair growth. You should try to allow the natural hair to grow for a few days before the visit.

U.S. Department of Health and Human Services, Office on Women's Health

http://www.womenshealth.gov

1-800-994-9662

TDD: 1-888-220-5446

Pelvic Exam. Your doctor might want to check to see if your ovaries are enlarged or swollen by the increased number of small cysts.

Blood Tests. Your doctor may check the androgen hormone and glucose (sugar) levels in your blood.

Vaginal Ultrasound (sonogram). Your doctor may perform a test that uses sound waves to take pictures of the pelvic area. It might be used to examine your ovaries for cysts and check the endometrium (en-do-MEE-tree-uhm) (lining of the womb). This lining may become thicker if your periods are not regular.

Q: How is PCOS treated?

A: Because there is no cure for PCOS, it needs to be managed to prevent problems. Treatment goals are based on your symptoms, whether or not you want to become pregnant, and lowering your chances of getting heart disease and diabetes. Many women will need a combination of treatments to meet these goals. Some treatments for PCOS include:

Lifestyle modification. Many women with PCOS are overweight or obese, which can cause health problems. You can help manage your PCOS by eating healthy and exercising to keep your weight at a healthy level. Healthy eating tips include:

- Limiting processed foods and foods with added sugars
- Adding more whole-grain products, fruits, vegetables, and lean meats to your diet

This helps to lower blood glucose (sugar) levels, improve the body's use of insulin, and normalize hormone levels in your body. Even a 10 percent loss in body weight can restore a normal period and make your cycle more regular.

Birth control pills. For women who don't want to get pregnant, birth control pills can:

- Control menstrual cycles
- Reduce male hormone levels
- Help to clear acne

Keep in mind that the menstrual cycle will become abnormal again if the pill is stopped. Women may also think about taking a pill that only has progesterone (proh-JES-tuh-rohn), like Provera, to control the menstrual cycle and reduce the risk of endometrial cancer (See "Does PCOS put women at risk for other health problems?"). But, progesterone alone does not help reduce acne and hair growth.

Diabetes medications. The medicine metformin (Glucophage) is used to treat type 2 diabetes. It has also been found to help with PCOS symptoms, though it isn't approved by the U.S. Food and Drug Administration (FDA) for this use. Metformin affects the way insulin controls blood glucose (sugar) and lowers testosterone production. It slows the growth of abnormal hair and, after a few months of use, may help ovulation to return. Recent research has shown metformin to have other positive effects, such as decreased body mass and improved cholesterol levels. Metformin will not cause a person to become diabetic.

Fertility medications. Lack of ovulation is usually the reason for fertility problems in women with PCOS. Several medications that stimulate ovulation can help women with PCOS become pregnant. Even so, other reasons for infertility in both the woman and man should be ruled out before

U.S. Department of Health and Human Services, Office on Women's Health

http://www.womenshealth.gov

1-800-994-9662

TDD: 1-888-220-5446

fertility medications are used. Also, some fertility medications increase the risk for multiple births (twins, triplets). Treatment options include:

- Clomiphene (KLOHM-uh-feen) (Clomid, Serophene) — the first choice therapy to stimulate ovulation for most patients.

- Metformin taken with clomiphene — may be tried if clomiphene alone fails. The combination may help women with PCOS ovulate on lower doses of medication.

- Gonadotropins (goe-NAD-oh-troe-pins) — given as shots, but are more expensive and raise the risk of multiple births compared to clomiphene.

Another option is in vitro fertilization (IVF). IVF offers the best chance of becoming pregnant in any given cycle. It also gives doctors better control over the chance of multiple births. But, IVF is very costly.

Surgery. "Ovarian drilling" is a surgery that may increase the chance of ovulation. It's sometimes used when a woman does not respond to fertility medicines. The doctor makes a very small cut above or below the navel (belly button) and inserts a small tool that acts like a telescope into the abdomen (stomach). This is called laparoscopy (lap-uh-RAHS-kuh-pee). The doctor then punctures the ovary with a small needle carrying an electric current to destroy a small portion of the ovary. This procedure carries a risk of developing scar tissue on the ovary. This surgery can lower male hormone levels and help with ovulation. But, these effects may only last a few months. This treatment doesn't help with loss of scalp hair or increased hair growth on other parts of the body.

page 4

Medicine for increased hair growth or extra male hormones. Medicines called anti-androgens may reduce hair growth and clear acne. Spironolactone (speer-on-oh-LAK-tone) (Aldactone), first used to treat high blood pressure, has been shown to reduce the impact of male hormones on hair growth in women. Finasteride (fin-AST-uhr-yd) (Propecia), a medicine taken by men for hair loss, has the same effect. Anti-androgens are often combined with birth control pills. These medications should not be taken if you are trying to become pregnant.

Before taking Aldactone, tell your doctor if you are pregnant or plan to become pregnant. Do not breastfeed while taking this medicine. Women who may become pregnant should not handle Propecia.

Other options include:

- Vaniqa (van-ik-uh) cream to reduce facial hair

- Laser hair removal or electrolysis to remove hair

- Hormonal treatment to keep new hair from growing

Other Treatments. Some research has shown that bariatric (weight loss) surgery may be effective in resolving PCOS in morbidly obese women. Morbid obesity means having a BMI of more than 40, or a BMI of 35 to 40 with an obesity-related disease. The drug troglitazone (troh-GLIT-uh-zohn) was shown to help women with PCOS. But, it was taken off the market because it caused liver problems. Similar drugs without the same side effect are being tested in small trials.

U.S. Department of Health and Human Services, Office on Women's Health

http://www.womenshealth.gov

1-800-994-9662

TDD: 1-888-220-5446

FREQUENTLY ASKED QUESTIONS

Researchers continue to search for new ways to treat PCOS. To learn more about current PCOS treatment studies, visit the clinicaltrials.gov Web site. Talk to your doctor about whether taking part in a clinical trial might be right for you.

Q: How does PCOS affect a woman while pregnant?

A: Women with PCOS appear to have higher rates of:

- Miscarriage
- Gestational diabetes
- Pregnancy-induced high blood pressure (preeclampsia)
- Premature delivery

Babies born to women with PCOS have a higher risk of spending time in a neonatal intensive care unit or of dying before, during, or shortly after birth. Most of the time, these problems occur in multiple-birth babies (twins, triplets).

Researchers are studying whether the diabetes medicine metformin can prevent or reduce the chances of having problems while pregnant. Metformin also lowers male hormone levels and limits weight gain in women who are obese when they get pregnant.

Metformin is an FDA pregnancy category B drug. It does not appear to cause major birth defects or other problems in pregnant women. But, there have only been a few studies of metformin use in pregnant women to confirm its safety. Talk to your doctor about taking metformin if you are pregnant or are trying to become pregnant. Also, metformin is passed through breastmilk. Talk with your doctor about metformin use if you are a nursing mother.

Q: Does PCOS put women at risk for other health problems?

A: Women with PCOS have greater chances of developing several serious health conditions, including life-threatening diseases. Recent studies found that:

- More than 50 percent of women with PCOS will have diabetes or pre-diabetes (impaired glucose tolerance) before the age of 40.
- The risk of heart attack is 4 to 7 times higher in women with PCOS than women of the same age without PCOS.
- Women with PCOS are at greater risk of having high blood pressure.
- Women with PCOS have high levels of LDL (bad) cholesterol and low levels of HDL (good) cholesterol.
- Women with PCOS can develop sleep apnea. This is when breathing stops for short periods of time during sleep.

Women with PCOS may also develop anxiety and depression. It is important to talk to your doctor about treatment for these mental health conditions.

Women with PCOS are also at risk for endometrial cancer. Irregular menstrual periods and the lack of ovulation cause women to produce the hormone estrogen, but not the hormone progesterone. Progesterone causes the endometrium (lining of the womb) to shed each month as a menstrual period. Without progesterone, the endometrium becomes thick, which can cause heavy or irregular bleeding. Over time, this can lead to endometrial hyperplasia, when the lining grows too much, and cancer.

U.S. Department of Health and Human Services, Office on Women's Health

http://www.womenshealth.gov

1-800-994-9662

TDD: 1-888-220-5446

Q: I have PCOS. What can I do to prevent complications?

A: If you have PCOS, get your symptoms under control at an earlier age to help reduce your chances of having complications like diabetes and heart disease. Talk to your doctor about treating all your symptoms, rather than focusing on just one aspect of your PCOS, such as problems getting pregnant. Also, talk to your doctor about getting tested for diabetes regularly. Other steps you can take to lower your chances of health problems include:

- Eating right
- Exercising
- Not smoking

Q: How can I cope with the emotional effects of PCOS?

A: Having PCOS can be difficult. You may feel:

- Embarrassed by your appearance
- Worried about being able to get pregnant
- Depressed

Getting treatment for PCOS can help with these concerns and help boost your self-esteem. You may also want to look for support groups in your area or online to help you deal with the emotional effects of PCOS. You are not alone and there are resources available for women with PCOS. ■

U.S. Department of Health and Human Services, Office on Women's Health

Appendix E: Sample of PCOS Basics Handout

PCOS Basics Handout

Polycystic Ovary Syndrome (PCOS) is an endocrine disorder that affects up to 10 percent of women. Common symptoms include irregular cycles, dark hair growth, weight gain, acne, infertility, recurrent miscarriage, and PMS.

PCOS is treated using medication, diet and exercise. Treatment is designed to help with weight loss, decrease insulin levels, balance hormones, improve fertility, regulate cycles, and decrease the risk of long-term health complications. If untreated, more than 50 percent of women with PCOS will develop impaired glucose tolerance (pre-diabetes) or type 2 diabetes by the age of 40, and they will have a 4-7 times greater risk for developing heart disease.

Nutritional counseling

We recommend following a healthy, well-balanced diet. Following a PCOS diet will help with weight loss and lowering insulin levels. *PCOSnutrition.com* offers free PCOS nutrition tips and information on the PCOS diet (pairing moderate complex carbohydrates/moderate protein and limiting simple sugar intake). We strongly recommend seeing a dietician for individual dietary counseling. Please let us know if you would like a referral to a dietician.

Psychological counseling

Counseling can be helpful in dealing with negative body image, eating disorders, weight gain, infertility, and depression. Please let us know if you would like a referral for psychological counseling.

Exercise

Exercise is very important. Exercise not only helps with weight reduction but it also helps the body better use insulin. High insulin levels tell your body to store fat. Correcting insulin resistance and losing weight will decrease your risk for long-term health complications such as diabetes, heart disease, and cancer.

Recommended Vitamins/Supplements

A daily multiple vitamin, Omega 3 fatty acids, Vitamin D3 1000-2000 i.u. per day, and Vitamin B12 1 cc injection 1 to 2 times per month.

The PCOS Workbook, Your Guide to Complete Physical and Emotional Health by Angela Grassi, MS, RD, LDN and Stephanie B Mattei, Psy.D. This is an excellent resource we highly recommend! It can be purchased at *www.PCOSnutrition.com* or on Amazon.com.

I've been Diagnosed with PCOS, Now What? A Guide to Thriving with PCOS by Lisa A. Borunda Conner, FNP-BC. This is a great little guide with loads of information about ways to manage PCOS and live a happier, healthier life. It can be purchased at our office, on Amazon.com, or on thrivingwithpcos.com.

PCOS Support Group

We offer a PCOS Education and Support Group on the first Tuesday of each month at 6 p.m. in our office.

Notes/Questions for my Healthcare Provider:

References

1. AACE Position Statement on Polycystic Ovary Syndrome. *EndocPract.* 2005;11(2):125-134.

2. Ashrafi M, Shelkhan F, Arabipoor A, et al. Gestational diabetes mellitus risk factors in women with polycystic ovary syndrome (PCOS). *European Journal of Obstetrics & Gynecology and Reproductive Biology.* Dec 2013;6:1-13.

3. Azziz R, Carmina E, Dewailly D, Diamanti-Kandarakis E, Escobar-Morreale HF, Futterweit W, et al. The Androgen Excess and PCOS Society criteria for the polycystic ovary syndrome: the complete task force report. *FertilSteril.* Feb 2009;91(2):456-488.

4. Azziz R, Woods KS, Reyna R, Key TJ, Knochenhauer ES, Yildiz BO. The prevalence and features of the polycystic ovary syndrome in an unselected population. *J ClinEndocrinolMetab.* Jun 2004;89(6):2745-27499.

5. Barbierei RL. Metformin for treatment of polycystic ovary syndrome. *Obstetrics and Gynecology.* 2003;101:785-793.

6. Carmina E. Diagnosis of polycystic ovary syndrome: from NIH criteria to ESHRE-ASRM guidelines. *Minervaginecologica.* Feb 2004;56(1): 1-6.

7. Diamanti-Kandarakis E, Spina G, Kouli C, et al. Increased endothelin-1 levels in women with polycystic ovary syndrome and the beneficial effect of metformin therapy. *J ClinEndocrinolMetab.* 2001;86:4666-4673.

8. Dunaif A, Finegood DT. Beta-cell dysfunction independent of obesity and glucose intolerance in the polcystic ovary syndrome. *J ClinEndocrinolMetab.* 1996;81:942-947.

9. Dunaif A, Segal KR, Futterweit W, Dobrjansky A. Profound peripheral insulin resistance, independent of obesity, in polycystic ovary syndrome. *Diabetes.* 1989;38:1165-1174.

10. Dunaif A, Wu X, Lee A, Diamanti-Kandarakis E. Defects in insulin receptor signaling in vivo in the polycystic ovary syndrome(PCOS). *Am J PhysiolEndocrinolMetub.* Aug 2001;281(2):E392-399.

11. Ehrmann DA, Barnes RB, Rosenfield RL, et al. Prevalence of impaired glucose tolerance and diabetes in women with polycystic ovary syndrome. *Diabetes Care.* Jan 1999;22(1):141-146.

12. Einhorn D, Reaven GM, Cobin RH, Ford E, Ganda OP, Handelsman Y, Hellman R, Jellinger PS, Kendall D, Drauss RM, Neufeld ND, Petak SM, Rodbard HW, Seibel JA, Smith DA, Wilson PW. ACE Position Statement on the Insulin Resistance Syndrome. *EndocrPract.* 2003;9(3):240-252.

13. Futterweit W. Pathophysiology of polycystic ovarian syndrome. In: Redmond GP, ed. Androgenic Disorders. New York: Raven Press, 1995: 77-166.

14. Glueck CJ, Papanna R, Wang P, Goldenberg N, Sieve-Smith L. Incidence and treatment of the metabolic syndrome in newly referred women with confirmed polycystic ovarian syndrome. *Metabolism.* 2003;5(2):908-915.

15. Gopal M, Duntley S, Uhles M, Attarian H. The role of obesity in the increased prevalence of obstructive sleep apnea syndrome in patients with polycystic ovarian syndrome. *Sleep Med.* Sep 2002;3(5):401-404.

16. Grassi A. The Dietician's Guide to Polycystic Ovary Syndrome. Luca Publishing: Haverford, PA., 2007:1-8.

17. Grassi A, Mattei S. The PCOS Workbook, your guide to complete physical and emotional health. Luca Publishing: Haverford, PA., 2009:21-28

18. Hamosh A. Polycystic ovary syndrome1: PCOS 1. *McKusick-Nathans Institute of Genetic Medicine. John Hopkins University School of Medicine.* Available at: http://omim.org/entry/184700. Retrieved 15 November 2011.

19. Hardiman P, Pillay OC, Atiomo W. Polycystic ovary syndrome and endometrial carcinoma. *Lancet.* May 24 2003;361(9371):1810-1812.

20. Knowler WC, Barrett, Connor E, Fowler SE, et al (Diabetes Prevention Program Research Group). Reduction in incidence of type 2 diabetes with lifestyle intervention or metformin. *N Engl J Med.* 2002;346:393-403.

21. Laws A, Reaven GM. Evidence for an independent relationship between insulin resistance and fasting plasma HDL-cholesterol, triglyceride and insulin concentrations. *J Int Med.* 1992;231:25-30.

22. Legro RS, Kunselman AR, Dodson WC, Dunaif A. Prevalence and predictors of risk for type 2 diabetes mellitus and impaired glucose tolerance in polycystic ovary syndrome: a prospective, controlled study in 254 affected women. *J ClinEndocrinolMetab.* Jan 1999;84(1):165-169.

23. Lillioja S, Mott DM, Spraul M, et al. Insulin resistance and insulin secretory dysfunction as precursors of non-insulin dependent diabetes mellitus. *N Engl J Med.* 1993;329:1988-1992.

24. Marsh K, Brand-Miller J. The optimal diet for women with polycystic ovary syndrome. *British Journal of Nutrition.* 2005;94:154-165.

25. McLaughlin T, Abbasi F, Kim HS, Lamendola C, Schaaf P, Reaven G. Relationship between insulin resistance, weight loss, and coronary heart disease risk in healthy, obese women. *Metabolism.* 2001;50:795-800.

26. Ogden CL, Yanovski SZ, Carroll MD, Flegal KM. The epidemiology of obesity. *Gastroenterology.* May 2007;132:2087-2102.

27. Ovalle F, Azziz R. Insulin resistance, polycystic ovary syndrome, and type 2 diabetes mellitus. *FertilSteril.* 2002;77:1095-1105.

28. Pontikis C, Yavropoulou, MP, Toulis KA, Kotsa K, Kazakos K, Papazisi A, et al. The incretin effect and secretionin obese and lean women with polycystic ovary syndrome: a pilot study. *J Womens Health.* Jun 2011;20(6):971-976.

29. PCOS Consensus Workshop Group. Rotterdam ESHRE/ASRM-Sponsored PCOS Consensus Workshop Group. Revised 2003 consensus on diagnostic criteria and long-term health risks related to polycystic ovary syndrome. *FertilSteril.* Jan 2004;81(1):19-25.

30. Sharma S, Nestler J. Prevention of cardiovascular disease and diabetes in women with PCOS: treatment with insulin sensitizers. *Best Pract Res ClinEndocrinolMetab.* 2006;20(2):245-260.

31. Sirmans SM, Pate KA. Epidemiology, diagnosis, and management of polycystic ovary syndrome. *Clinical Epidemiology.* Oct 2014;181:195-199.

32. Toulis KA, Goulis DG, Farmakiotis D, Georgopoulos NA, Katsikis I, Tarlatzis BC, et al. Adiponectin levels in women with polycystic ovary syndrome: a systematic review and a meta-analysis. *Hum Reprod Update.* May-Jun 2009;15(3):297-307.

33. Tran N, Hunter S, Yankowitz J. Oral hypoglycemic agents in pregnancy. *Obstetrical and Gynecological Survey.* 2004;59(6),456-463.

34. Tuomilehto J, Lindstrom J, Eriksson JG, et al. Prevention of type 2 diabetesby changes in lifestyle among subjects with impaired glucose tolerance. *N Engl J Med.* 2001;344:1343-1350.

35. US Dept of Health and Human Services, Office on Women's Health. Polycystic Ovary Syndrome FAQ. Available at: www.womenshealth.gov. Retrieved 15 September 2011.

36. Warram JH, Martin BC, Krowlewski AS, et al. Slow glucose removal rate and hyperinsulinemia precede the development of type II diabetes in the off-spring of the diabetic parents. *Ann Intern Med.* 1990;113:909-915.

Made in the USA
Columbia, SC
28 June 2019